The Miracle RESULTS of FASTING

DAVE WILLIAMS

The Miracle RESULTS OF FASTING

YOUR SECRET WEAPON IN SPIRITUAL WARFARE

THE MIRACLE RESULTS OF FASTING

Copyright ©1997 by David R. Williams

First Printing 1997

ISBN 0-938020-50-1

Published by

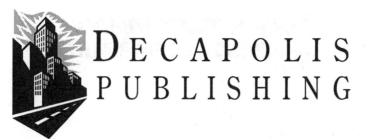

DECAPOLIS PUBLISHING

BOOKS BY DAVID R. WILLIAMS

AIDS Plague
Beauty of Holiness
Christian Job Hunter's Handbook
Desires of Your Heart
Depression, Cave of Torment
Finding Your Ministry & Gifts
Genuine Prosperity
Getting To Know Your Heavenly Father
Grand Finale Revival
Growing Up in Our Father's Family
How to Be a High Performance Believer in Low Octane Days
Laying On of Hands
Lonely in the Midst of a Crowd
The New Life . . . The Start of Something Wonderful
La Nueva Vida (The New Life . . . SPANISH)
Pacesetting Leadership
The Pastor's Pay
Patient Determination
Revival Power of Music
Remedy for Worry and Tension
Secret of Power With God
Seven Signposts on the Road to Spiritual Maturity
Slain in the Spirit — Real or Fake?
Somebody Out There Needs You
Success Principles From the Lips of Jesus
Supernatural Soulwinning
Thirty-Six Minutes with the Pastor
Tongues and Interpretation
Understanding Spiritual Gifts

Special Thanks

I would like to give thanks to our editorial staff and team: Linda Teagan, Julie Feldpausch, Betsy Garza, Cristel Phelps, Heather Gleason, Sue Heyboer, Pam Mandwee, Joe Rabideau and Eldon Langworthy. Thanks also to Michael Tomanica for artwork. And special thanks to my wonderful wife Mary Jo Williams for her work, support, and encouragement. Thank you all for your many hours of assistance and speedy, hard work in completing this book.

CONTENTS

Read This First 11

Intensified Revelation 15

What is Fasting? 19

Different Kinds of Fasting 25

Purposes and Rewards of Fasting 35

Getting Into Position 43

Dave Roever's Experience 47

Fasting at Any Age 51

Your Rewards For Fasting 55

Defeating Leviathan 59

Leviathan's Tail 69

Promised Benefits From Isaiah 58 73

Choose Your Plan, and Take Action 85

READ THIS FIRST

I just returned from a retirement banquet in honor of my dear friend, Loren Triplett. Loren served eight years as the director of foreign missions for his denomination, overseeing an annual budget of nearly $120,000,000. Loren has stepped down from his high position, but he certainly isn't stepping out of the picture. He has plans — missionary plans.

Loren is an impressive fellow. During his time as director of foreign missions, the number of overseas church members and adherents grew from 16 million to 25 million. The number of foreign national ministers increased 48 percent. To top that off, when Loren assumed the directorship in 1989, we had missionaries in 86 nations. After just eight years of Loren's leadership, we now have mission efforts in 148 nations of the world. Now, *that's* an achievement.

Loren Triplett is one of the godliest men I've ever had the privilege of knowing. I have witnessed his "breakneck" achievements over the years. Fifty years ago as a young pastor, he felt called to serve on the mission field, and in just one day raised 100 percent of his missionary term support. In a miracle camp meeting, God moved on his listener's hearts, and people stormed Loren and his wife, Milly, with money, diamonds, and whatever else they could give. Typically, a missionary today needs eighteen months to raise a full term of support.

How has Loren accomplished so much in such a short time? What is his secret? Ask the people who know him. You will learn that Loren has lived a "**fasted**" life.

You may not understand the word "**fast**" yet, but by the time you finish reading this book, you will. And you will have a burning desire to practice fasting yourself because of the many benefits it brings to your life; benefits such as these:

- ♦ Deliverance from bad habits
- ♦ Revelations from God
- ♦ Speedily answered prayers
- ♦ Constant supply of your needs
- ♦ Rejuvenation of your health and vitality
- ♦ A longer life
- ♦ Loss of unwanted weight

- Slowing down the aging process
- Elimination of body toxins
- Elimination of food allergy sources
- Clearing of acne and other dermatological problems
- Defeating sinus and mucus problems
- Normalizing your blood pressure
- Helping to keep your arteries young
- Healthy cholesterol levels
- Assistance in curing mental and emotional disorders
- Giving you increased energy levels
- Bringing your body into spiritual subjection
- Breaking demonic forces

In fact, according to Ronald G. Cridland, M.D., **"fasting can save your life!"**

There are always critics who sneer, no matter what I teach. And certainly there are critics of the practice of fasting. They call it "starvation." This is nonsense.

"The most popular criticisms of fasting are written by people who never missed a meal in their lives."

—*A. Rabogliati, A.M., M.D., F.R.C.S.*

This book is a written combination of a message I preached in 1986, as well as a fresh revelation from the Holy Spirit to my heart. I urgently wanted to

get this message into your hands. We pressed ourselves to complete this task on time. My goal is to
motivate you and inspire you to live a fasted life.
Then, you, too, will see amazing advances in your
life, so that people at *your* banquet of honor will
say, as they did at Loren Triplett's, "How did he do
that?"

In this book, I'm going to share with you an important, life-changing message on fasting for a desired result. To choose to deny yourself food in or-
der to achieve some spiritual or physical benefit may
seem crazy. However, fasting for a desired result is
a biblical precept long practiced by those who have
sought God for miracles.

We will study about what fasting is, the different types of fasting, the purpose of fasting, and the
proper attitude for fasting. You will be excited to
learn the awesome rewards of fasting. Also, I will
share with you some revelation about the most sinister, evil, dangerous, demonic spirit that could ever
be loosed against a human being or a ministry. In
the Bible, he's simply called, "Leviathan." I will also
show you how you can avoid the sweeping tail of
Leviathan.

It's an exciting message. Happy fasting!

— Dave Williams
Springfield, Missouri
November 1997

CHAPTER 1

INTENSIFIED REVELATION

What if *you* could do something that would bring amazing blessings to your life, would cost you nothing, and would hurt no one? Blessings like:

♦ Deliverance from bad habits
♦ Revelations from God
♦ Divine Protection
♦ Quickly answered prayers
♦ Speedy return of health
♦ A constant supply of your needs

Would you like to receive blessings like these? You can. Fasting will help you receive these benefits.

Fasting, which is abstaining from food, was practiced by great men and women in the Bible. I found it was also a regular practice of the most powerful contemporary ministers and ministries. And, I discovered that fasting can catapult a person's life, work, or ministry years ahead of schedule.

I fasted quite a bit in the early years of my ministry, and *that* is when I began to discover its astonishing value and benefits. Prior to that, I thought fasting was sort of an "iffy" thing. You can fast if you want to, but you don't have to. Mostly, I didn't want to. But when I really began to study what the Bible said about fasting, I decided to do it. I spent three days in total abstinence. I ate no food at all.

After the three days without food, I went into a prolonged "Daniel Fast," where I ate no pleasant food. Daniel said, "I ate no pleasant bread." That means he didn't eat cake, bread, or meat. He procured his protein from other sources. I stayed on that fast for a couple of months and found I was drawn closer to God; I discovered an intensified revelation of Him. In fact, during that time of fasting, I received more revelation knowledge than I had ever received in my whole combined Christian experience. And, as an added benefit, I shed fifty pounds of unsightly fat!

God spoke to me. He said, "Dave, as a result of this fasting, I am advancing your ministry by ten years."

In other words, what would normally have taken me ten years to accomplish only took me a matter of months! These benefits were the direct result of the concentrated, intensified power of God that was working in my life through fasting!

Then I read about other ministers like D. L. Moody, Charles Finney, and Charles Spurgeon; those who rose out of obscurity and became great soul winners. I learned that they all practiced fasting *regularly.* And the results they experienced were world changing.

"Therefore also now, saith the Lord, turn ye even to me with all your heart, and with fasting, and with weeping, and with mourning."

— Joel 2:12

CHAPTER 2

WHAT IS FASTING?

Fasting always involves abstaining from food. Some types of fasting may involve abstaining from only certain types of food, but it *always* involves abstinence. Food is not bad. We must eat to live, but our appetites can run out of control. Too much of even a good thing can lead us to be "out of control." Anything out of control, whether it's an automobile or a person, is dangerous.

Fasting humbles the soul before God; it denies and masters the appetite; it manifests an earnest desire to seek God; it helps in giving us power over demonic oppression; and it aids in prayer.

"Is not this the fast that I have chosen? To loose the bands of wickedness, to undo the heavy burdens, and to let the oppressed go free, and that ye break every yoke that is bondage?

Is it not to deal thy bread to the hungry, and that thou bring the poor that are cast out to thy house? When thou seest the naked, that thou cover him; and that thou hide not thyself from thine own flesh?

Then shall thy light break forth as the morning, and thine health shall spring forth speedily: and thy righteousness shall go before thee; the glory of the Lord shall be thy rereward.

Then shalt thou call, and the Lord shall answer; thou shalt cry, and he shall say, Here I am. If thou take away from the midst of thee the yoke, the putting forth of the finger, and speaking vanity;

And if thou draw out thy soul to the hungry, and satisfy the afflicted soul; then shall thy light rise in obscurity, and thy darkness be as the noonday:

And the Lord shall guide thee continually, and satisfy thy soul in drought, and make fat thy bones: and thou shalt be like a watered garden, and like a spring of water, whose waters fail not.

> *And they that shall be of thee, shall build the old waste places: thou shalt raise up the foundations of many generations; and thou shalt be called, The repairer of the breach, The restorer of paths to dwell in."*
>
> — *Isaiah 58:6-12*

"Is not this the fast that I have chosen?" God, through the prophet Isaiah, enumerates some of the benefits of fasting. If you have a nicotine habit or any other addiction, God is going to show you how fasting can cure you of it. You can be delivered from the things that have held you in bondage for years, but for some reason haven't been able to shake.

> *"Then was Jesus led up of the Spirit into the wilderness to be tempted of the devil. And when he had fasted forty days and forty nights, he was afterward an hungred. And when the tempter came to him, he said, If thou be the Son of God, command that these stones be made bread. But he answered and said, It is written, Man shall not live by bread alone, but by every word that proceedeth out of the mouth of God.*
>
> — *Matthew 4:1-4*

> *"And when they were come to the multitude, there came to him a certain man, kneeling down to him, and saying, Lord, have mercy on my son: for he is lunatic, and sore vexed: for ofttimes he falleth into the fire, and*

> oft into the water. And I brought him to thy
> disciples, and they could not cure him.
>
> Then Jesus answered and said, O faithless
> and perverse generation, how long shall I be
> with you? how long shall I suffer you? bring
> him hither to me. And Jesus rebuked the devil;
> and he departed out of him: and the child was
> cured from that very hour.
>
> Then came the disciples to Jesus apart, and
> said, Why could we not cast him out? And
> Jesus said unto them, Because of your
> unbelief: for verily I say unto you, If ye have
> faith as a grain of mustard seed, ye shall say
> unto this mountain, Remove hence to yonder
> place; and it shall remove; and nothing will
> be impossible unto you. Howbeit this kind
> goeth not out but by prayer and fasting.
> — Matthew 17:14-21

Do you know that every Christian is expected
to fast? When Jesus taught about fasting, He said,
"*When* you fast, be not as the hypocrites," (Matthew
6:16). He didn't say, "*If* you choose to fast." He said,
"*When* you fast."

Fasting was *not* an option. Yet there were no
harsh regulations or legalistic, regimented rules for
fasting. It was left to the discretion of each individual. However, historical records show us that in
the beginning stages of church history, there was a
regular time of fasting. These times of fasting were

called by the church leaders and were typically on Wednesdays and Fridays.

More doctors, especially Spirit-filled ones, are beginning to recognize the value of fasting. I went to a Christian doctor because I had an annoying allergy. I said, "Doctor, I've got this sinus difficulty." He looked at me, and the first thing he asked was, "Have you tried fasting?"

"Have I what?" I sputtered. "Come on, don't you have a pill or something that can clear it up?"

Well, I tried his suggestion. And through fasting and proper nutrition, the allergies that plagued me for two decades were wiped out. It is great to enter the summer and fall seasons without sneezing, wheezing, and itching.

Later in this book you will learn more about the physical benefits of fasting, but I think it's marvelous that doctors are beginning to recognize the value of this biblical practice. I would recommend that before you go on a prolonged fast, you visit your family doctor. Some people have medical conditions that should be checked before they go on a prolonged fast. However, I believe every Christian, in some way or another, can participate in a fast.

"And when they had ordained them elders in every church, and had prayed with fasting, they commended them to the Lord, on whom they believed."

— *Acts 14:23*

CHAPTER 3

DIFFERENT KINDS OF FASTING

What are the different types of fasting? Basically there are two types. One is the corporate fast; the other is the personal fast. There is power in both kinds of fasting.

CORPORATE FASTING

Corporate fasting is called by the leadership — either the spiritual leadership or the governmental leadership. In 2 Chronicles, Chapter 20, Jehosaphat, the king of Judah, proclaimed a fast because he was seeking a word of wisdom from the Lord. He wanted to know what to do about some enemies that were preparing to invade his land.

Judah did not have the resources available to fend off these enemies, so Jehosaphat and his people sought the Lord in fasting, prayer, and praise. God gave a word of wisdom almost immediately when they began to fast. The word of wisdom came, "Stand still, and see the salvation of the Lord." As God's people fasted, their enemies tore each other apart. God's people were spared because their leader called them together corporately and said, "Everybody fast."

In Jonah, Chapter 3, Jonah went down to the city of Ninevah and said, "Judgment is coming." The heathen leader of Ninevah believed the prophet of God and called the entire city to a time of corporate fasting to show an inward repentance. Everyone in Ninevah, including the children and the animals, fasted. As a result, God said, "I'm not going to send the judgment I had planned for Ninevah."

Something special happens when a spiritual leader or a governmental leader calls a corporate fast.

The book of Esther relates another miracle result of fasting. A serious danger to God's people was imminent. There was a man, Haman, in the king's cabinet stirring up trouble against the Jews in the land where Esther and Mordecai lived. He was planning to initiate a serious persecution against the Jewish people to kill them all. So, Mordecai called for a corporate fast. Do you know what happened? The tables turned on the wicked man who designed the sinister plot, and he himself was hanged on the gallows he had prepared for the Jews. God always protects His people when they seek Him with fasting and prayer.

Have you ever faced enemy oppression? Sometimes the enemy comes as a "holy angel of light." He comes as a wolf in sheep's clothing. He doesn't come and say, "Hi, I'm a wolf." He dresses like a sheep, smells like a sheep, talks like a sheep, but on the inside, he is a wolf. God can turn the tables on that wolf. He can help you overcome oppression and give you victory in every situation through fasting and prayer.

I wonder what would have happened if the principle behind this miracle in the book of Esther had been applied before the Holocaust in World War II? What if, beforehand, nations were called together for fasting and prayer? History may have been different.

Fathers may call their households to a time of family fasting. A pastor may call his church to a time of corporate fasting. In Acts, Chapter 13, the leaders called for a corporate fast before selecting and ordaining elders.

Sometimes, we take too lightly the ordination of new ministers. Instead of fasting and praying, we stuff ourselves at a banquet before the service, and, still burping our beef, we lay our hands on the new ministers and pray that God will bless their ministries. Candidly, we can't really seek God's presence or direction — we are too stuffed with food; we are thinking about a nap!

I believe there should always be prayer and fasting involved in selecting church leaders. Still, occasionally we select a "Judas." Even Jesus had a Judas. But, if there has been corporate prayer and fasting *before* the laying on of hands and the sending out of new leadership, there won't be very many "Judases." Corporate fasting and prayer is scriptural and very important.

I have discovered that when a church begins to corporately fast and pray, "impurities" begin to surface. That's when attitude problems and character flaws are revealed. There have been times when I hated corporate fasting because it seemed like everyone got so irritable. But when the impurities begin to surface, the Holy Spirit blows them away. *The benefit of fasting often comes after the fast has been completed.*

I'm ashamed of myself that, as a pastor, I haven't called more church-wide fasts. I want to begin every new year with forty days of fasting in our church. Forty is the Hebrew number for purification and preparation. That is why in Noah's day the waters broke loose for forty days and forty nights. It was the time required for purification. God purified the earth.

Corporate fasting purifies the collective body. Personal fasting purifies the individual body.

PERSONAL FASTING

Personal fasting is the other type of fasting. It is still abstaining from food or from certain foods, but it is done by just one individual. Moses fasted forty days. David fasted often, and he was called a man after God's own heart. He fasted while interceding for a friend (see Psalm 35:13). Nehemiah fasted while seeking guidance from God. Daniel fasted often and received many revelations and visions from God. Jesus began His public ministry with forty days of fasting.

John the Baptist fasted regularly. He abstained from food other than locusts and honey. Would you care to go on one of those kinds of fasts? "Grass-hoppers and honey, anybody? Sorry, locusts are out of season!" What a menu!

Anna, the prophetess, fasted often in the temple. Historical records say she lived to be between 106 to 110 years old. How would you like to live to be 110? I don't mean a doddering, weak, old age, but an old age filled with energy and vitality. You need to fast. You're not going to do it living on junk food.

When you go into a personal fast, your body begins to purify itself of poisons. We put some stupid things into our bodies like caffeine, nicotine, and chocolate. Preservatives, additives, and all kinds of toxins could be in your liver right now, just waiting to disease you.

Dr. Dean Ornish says that after fasting just 12 hours, toxins will begin to leave your system. We all have a unique, built-in repair system. When you fast just 12 hours, your body will begin the reparative process. The poisons that are damaging your system will begin to come out. That is why your tongue gets a coat on it when you fast, and you get a terrible taste in your mouth. You say, "My mouth tastes awful, and my tongue has a coat on it." That "coat" is the evidence that the poisons are beginning to come out of your body through fasting and prayer. I tell people that when they are fasting, make sure they have one of those little breath spray bottles handy.

NOTE: Please don't take this next section as a medical recommendation. It is not my purpose to give medical advice or recommend a course of action from a medical standpoint. I'm just relating an historic case on the physical benefits one man derived from fasting.

I remember a man we all called, "Pa." When he was 81 years old, his doctor diagnosed him with cancer. The prognosis was, "If you don't have immediate surgery, you'll die within a matter of weeks. If you do have surgery, you still might die, but there would be a chance we could save your life." He faced a choice: have the surgery and perhaps die or don't have the surgery and surely die.

"Pa" decided not to have the surgery. He wasn't a particularly religious man, but he went home and started on a strange kind of fast. He began to abstain from certain meats and ate just boiled food, like rhubarb and fruits and vegetables.

"Pa" lived for 16 more "fruitful" and healthy years. He died at the age of 97, but he *didn't* die of cancer. Fasting restored his health, and it can restore yours, too.

As you can see from these examples, corporate fasting and personal fasting are both biblical and beneficial. You can get miracle results from fasting.

"And it came to pass, when I heard these words, that I sat down and wept, and mourned certain days, and fasted, and prayed before the God of heaven."

— Nehemiah 1:4

WHY FAST?
by Dr. Bill Bright

Fasting is a primary means of restoration. By humbling us, fasting releases the Holy Spirit to do His revival work within us. This takes us deeper into the Christlife and gives us a greater awareness of God's reality and presence in our lives.

- Fasting reduces the power of self so that the Holy Spirit can do a more intense work within us.
- Fasting helps to purify us spiritually.
- Fasting increases our spiritual reception by quieting our minds and emotions.
- Fasting brings a yieldedness, even a holy brokenness, resulting in an inner calm and self-control.
- Fasting renews spiritual vision.
- Fasting inspires determination to follow God's revealed plan for your life.

— *Bill Bright, Adapted from* **The Coming Revival: America's Call to Fast, Pray and Seek God's Face**
©1995 Bill Bright. New Life Publications.

"But thou, when thou fastest, anoint thine head, and wash thy face; That thou appear not unto men to fast, but unto thy Father which is in secret: and thy Father, which seeth in secret, shall reward thee openly."

— Matthew 6:17-18

CHAPTER 4

PURPOSES AND REWARDS OF FASTING

What is the purpose of fasting? Purposes may differ. Biblical purposes include:

♦ Increased prayer power
♦ Divine protection
♦ Physical healing
♦ Emotional or relational healing
♦ Intercession for friends
♦ Repentance and sorrow
♦ Seeking God for guidance or direction

Your personal purposes for fasting may be different than the church's corporate purposes; but in nature, fasting serves basically the same purpose: it gets us into a position to receive from God.

Someone might say, "Well, aren't you trying to twist God's arm by fasting?" No! I am just trying to get my spirit, mind, and body into a position to receive whatever God has for me.

I am quite certain that my own ministry was advanced by several years as a result of fasting and prayer. I know your life, your business, or your ministry can be advanced at a supernatural rate if you fast and pray. The mercury in your spiritual "thermometer" will shatter the top as His Spirit flows into you and He fills your life with purpose and power.

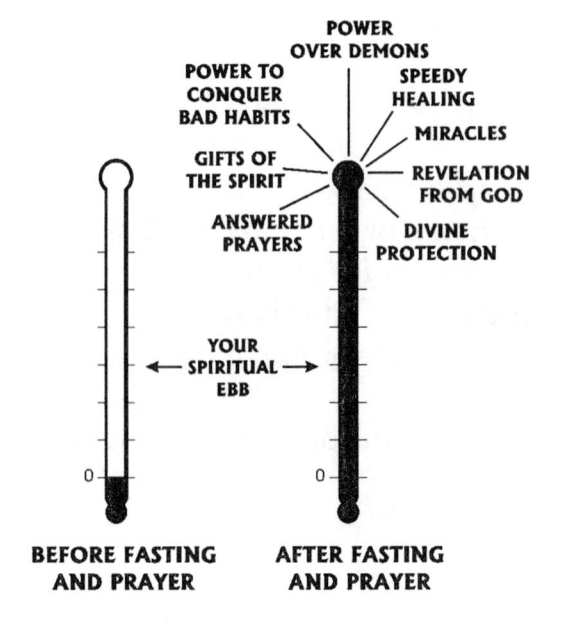

YOUR "POWER THERMOMETER"

What does fasting do? It seems to intensify or concentrate God's power in our lives. We're not trying to twist God's arm. I have heard immature people who say, "I'm going to fast until either God answers my prayer or I die." It turns out to be more of a hunger strike than a fast — a hunger strike against God. Well, that is immature. We don't fast to get God to do something; we fast to bring ourselves into a position where we're increasingly in tune with Him, so we can receive what He wants us to have.

God wants us healthy! God wants us to have good things! "Beloved, I wish above all things that thou mayest prosper and be in health, even as thy soul prospereth," (3 John 2). God wants to guide us continually! God wants to protect us and our property! The discipline of fasting will put us into position to receive these blessings. It intensifies or concentrates God's power at work in our lives.

Jesus said there's a certain kind of demon that goes out only by fasting and prayer. When the disciples asked, "Why couldn't we drive it out?" Jesus answered in Matthew 17:21, "This kind goeth not out but by fasting and prayer." The disciples already had God's power working in their lives, but Jesus pointed out that their power would be intensified by fasting and prayer.

Does fasting produce faith? No, it doesn't actually generate faith — only the Word of God can produce faith. But fasting does heighten and sharpen the faith we already possess. Fasting puts a razor's edge on your faith to get you into a position to receive whatever it is you need.

What is the proper attitude for fasting? Let's see what the Bible has to say:

> *"Moreover, when ye fast, be not, as the hypocrites of a sad countenance: for they disfigure their faces, that they may appear unto men to fast."*
>
> *— Matthew 6:16a*

Notice, the hypocrite's true motivation is wanting to *appear* to be fasting. That's why he fasts. He wants to appear to be a spiritual "big-shot."

It sounds something like this:

"Hey, do you want to go to lunch today?"

The hypocrite responds with a spiritually superior look on his face, "Oh, no! I'm ... fasting."

"Oooh, you're so spiritual!" is what he longs to hear.

When that happens, he just received his reward. All the reward he ever got for that time of fasting is that somebody said to him, "Oh, you're so spiritual."

If someone invites you to lunch, and you accept, I can guarantee that God is not going to be telling you to fast on that day. I've actually had people invited to a meal come and say they can't eat because they are fasting. I believe that is a false motivation, to appear to men to be fasting. It isn't wrong for people to know you are fasting, but if you tell them in a way that brings attention to yourself, in essence you are saying, "Look at me. Look how spiritual I am." That is false motivation.

Yet, people are going to know you are fasting when we call a church-wide, corporate fast. If somebody asks, "Do you want to go out to lunch," simply say, "No, thanks. Today is one of my days." You haven't lost your reward because your motivation is not to be seen of men. Your motivation is to receive a reward from your heavenly Father.

Remember what Jesus said about true fasting motivation:

> *"Verily I say unto you, they have their reward. But thou, when thou fastest, anoint*

> thine head, and wash thy face; that thou
> appear not unto men to fast, but unto thy
> Father which is in secret: and thy Father, which
> seeth in secret, shall **reward you** openly."
> — *Matthew 6: 16b - 18*

There is a reward in fasting.

This is one of the major keys of fasting that most have missed. You must focus on the reward of fasting. What reward are you seeking? Well, that has to be determined *before* you begin to fast. In Ezra, the Jews determined that their reward was going to be protection during a journey for their families, their little ones, and their possessions. They decided to fast and clearly stated, "Lord, this is the reward we want. We want divine protection." God gave them their reward. They kept their eyes focused on the reward, not on their hunger.

A terrible way to fast is to make the decision, "I'm going to fast today," then you watch someone eating their lunch and think, "Oh, that sure looks good! I wish I could eat, but I'm fasting. Poor me, I'm so hungry!" When you focus on your deprivation instead of focusing on the expected reward, fasting is a tough job.

When you focus on the reward, whatever reward you have asked for in secret, the Bible says your heavenly Father will reward you openly. Do you want to be delivered from bad habits? Do you want to be delivered from demonic oppression? I know people who have been depressed all their lives. They have never learned the secret of fasting. Do you want to learn the secret of breaking the yoke of depression? Learn the secret of fasting, prayer, and praise. Then watch as all your yokes are broken.

But you must determine the reward first. You are not buying the reward; you are just *expecting* the reward. "Lord, this is the reward I want. I want a deeper relationship with You. I want to have protection for my family. I want to have salvation for my loved ones." I know a man whose wife was not saved, so he fasted for her salvation. I don't remember how long he fasted. I just know his wife came speedily to the church and accepted Christ right there in front of the whole congregation. Do you want to see supernatural things happen? Get involved in fasting, and expect the reward.

If you are fasting, expect a reward. If you pray, expect answers. There is too much "slot-machine religion" in the church today. Some think, "Well, I'll put my silver dollar in and hope my lucky number comes up." That is fatalism. That's a "que sera, sera" attitude. That is not God. God says to expect something from what you do. Expect answers to your prayers. Expect reward from your fasting. I expect big rewards. I have my rewards listed out first. If I'm going to fast, there's going to be a reward involved.

Fasting is one Christian discipline that helps us spiritually, mentally, emotionally, relationally, financially, and physically. It even helps your memory, but not for the first few days. For the first few days, your appetite is clamoring for food. During the first few days, you might have a headache. On a complete fast where you drink only distilled water, you may experience headaches, dizziness, weakness, trembling, abdominal pains, and nausea. Dr. Dean Ornish said this is actually a result of poisons coming out of your body. Don't worry about it. After a few days, your body will finally catch on; you're not going to feed it. Your stomach actually quits producing acids, and you will lose your screaming appetite.

Remember, concentrate on the reward, not the way your body responds to the fast. Always fast for a desired reward, and God will reward you!

CHAPTER 5

GETTING INTO POSITION

How do we get into a position to receive the desired reward? What are the regulations for fasting? Actually, there are no clear regulations. It is not to be a legalistic, regimented type of practice, although there may be a regular time or special time of fasting.

James Hamill, who was the pastor at First Assembly of God in Memphis, Tennessee, found a lump on his body and went to his physician to have it diagnosed. It was cancer. One of the church leaders came before the congregation and said, "Our pastor has cancer — terminal cancer. We don't want to lose him. We had better fast and pray that God will answer our prayer and heal him." It's amazing how quickly God answers when people fast and pray.

Pastor Hamill's congregation began to fast and pray. In just a few days, the lump disappeared. He went back to his physician, and the doctor ran all kinds of tests. There was no trace of cancer anywhere in his body, and he went on for many more fruitful years at First Assembly in Memphis. In fact, after that experience he wrote a book called *Pastor to Pastor,* a book to help and encourage pastors. How did this miracle happen? The whole church got into a position to receive rewards from God, and God intensified His healing power through fasting and prayer.

Do you need your family saved? Children protected? Wisdom? Anointing? Favor? Healing? Do you have an overwhelming problem? Have you failed in the past and want to succeed in the future? There are many promises for people who fast.

Christians and non-Christians alike can have similar physical and mental benefits of fasting. However, as Christians, we are able to have the added benefit of positioning ourselves to receive not only physical and mental benefits but also to receive spiritual advantages. Perhaps you are reading this and have never committed your life to Christ. You can do that right now.

If you want to make a decision to accept Jesus Christ as your Savior, you need to know and believe that He died on the cross, and He rose from the dead. Why did He die? Because of you, because of me, because we've all sinned and fallen short of His standards.

You can have the opportunity of eternal life as a child of God just by saying, "Yes!" to Jesus. He loves you. No matter how badly you have failed and fallen into sin, if you repent and turn from that sin, you will have a home in heaven forever.

Pray this prayer with me now:

Dear God,

I come to You in the name of Jesus. Your Word says that if I turn to You, You will not cast me out but will take me in just as I am. I thank You, God, for that. I believe Jesus died on the cross for me, that He was raised from the dead, and I confess Him as my Lord. Please forgive my sins, and give me a new start beginning right now. Thank You, Lord!

Amen

If you have just prayed this prayer, write to me, and I will send you a free copy of my book, **The New Life . . . The Start of Something Wonderful**. Over 2.5 million people now have this book.

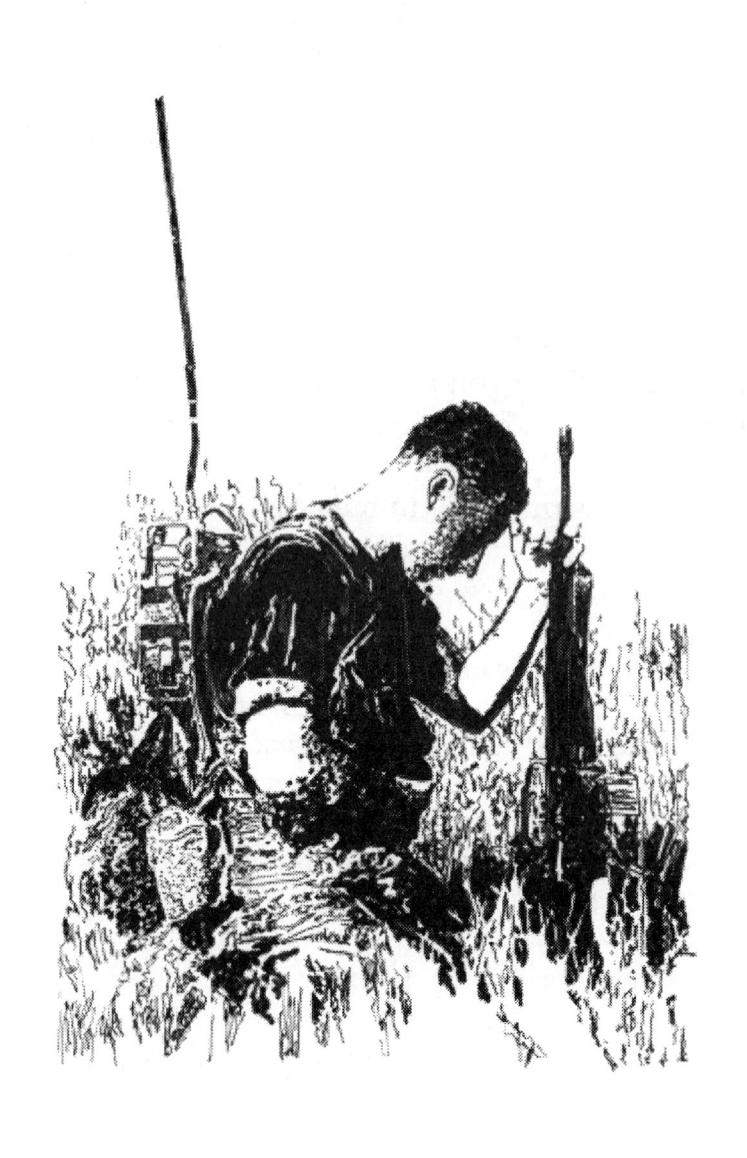

CHAPTER 6

DAVE ROEVER'S EXPERIENCE

Evangelist Dave Roever, a dear friend of mine, recently told me of his amazing experience of fasting for forty days. It miraculously changed his life and advanced his ministry call to Vietnam by virtual light years.

Dave served in the U.S. Navy's special forces during the Vietnam war. In 1969, while preparing to throw a white phosphorous hand grenade, a sniper fired at Dave, hitting the grenade, causing it to explode in his hand. Dave was burned beyond recognition. Sixty pounds of his flesh was burned away.

By a miracle of God, he survived. Though he was physically scarred for life, there are no scars in his spirit or emotions. God has put a love in Dave's heart for the Vietnamese people, as well as a dream to reach that communist nation for Christ.

Over the years, after many surgeries, Dave gained quite a bit of excess weight. Doctors told him he wouldn't live to be fifty years old because of his original injuries and subsequent treatments.

When he turned fifty, God began to move on Dave's heart to fast for forty days. A new direction was about to divinely unfold in Dave's life, but he needed to prepare himself.

For thirty days, he consumed nothing but distilled water. Amazingly, after the first few days, his body was filled with energy and vitality. His excess weight seemed to melt away, not by the fire of a white phosphorous grenade this time but by the fire of the cleansing power of fasting. His system was being cleansed. In fact, after a week or so, he found that he needed to use no deodorant. Even his perspiration had a clean, fresh, smell.

After thirty days, Dave started drinking diluted juices in preparation for breaking the fast. For ten days, he still ate no food, only weak juices.

Dave testifies he received divine guidance and a loving closeness to Jesus like he had never experienced before. Also, this time of fasting launched Dave onto a nutritional plan that helped him shed over 110 pounds. His life and ministry now have a fresh start and a new vitality. His time of fasting catapulted his life into a greater realization of God's love, care, guidance, and desire to reach the lost and hurting people of the world.

Dave has always had a heart for the Vietnamese children whose grandfathers were killed during the war. Since the fast, a great miracle of supply occurred. The Japanese government gave $1.1 million worth of children's clothes to Dave Roever's ministry. Subsequently, Dave distributed the clothes to poor Vietnamese children. Further, God has given Dave favor with the Vietnamese government, and he will likely be the first evangelist to conduct an open air crusade in that once war-torn country.

One major church leader had a vision of millions of Vietnamese people coming to Jesus Christ through Dave Roever's ministry. It will likely become a reality before the year 2000.

In the 60's and 70's, we tried to save Vietnam with M-16's and failed. Now Vietnam will be saved, not with an M-16 but with John 3:16!

The question is, would all the opportunities have opened up to Dave Roever if he had not fasted forty days? No one knows for sure, but Dave wouldn't trade the experience for anything in the world. Since his time of fasting, his ministry has advanced in God's will, and Dave is receiving heaven's direction with an astonishing clarity.

CHAPTER 7

FASTING AT ANY AGE

Mr. "B," seventy years old, had struggled with several medical problems most of his life. He had been hospitalized many times, five times for asthma alone. He could find no relief until a brilliant young doctor suggested an extended fast.

Mr. "B" decided to try fasting. It was difficult at first. He seemed to be worse as he struggled to breathe, yet no drugs were administered, and he remained under the constant supervision of his physician.

After only six days, his enlarged prostate had shrunk to the size of a young man's. He was able to urinate as freely as a boy.

He continued to fast. His sinuses cleared; his breathing became normal. On the thirty-sixth day of his fast, a miracle occurred. He regained permanent hearing in his deaf ear. After 42 days, he resumed eating gradually, beginning with diluted juices.

Another surprise, his libido returned. He was no longer impotent. After almost seventy years of suffering, in 42 days he was miraculously healed!

MORE FASTING RESULTS

Roy White is 106 years old and looks like he's 60. He fasts four times a year for seven days and does progressive weight training three times a week.

At the age of 70, Martin Cornica was playing a championship tennis game with much younger players — and winning. His secret? Regular fasting! He said he feels like a 20 year old out there on the court.

"Fasting is simply wonderful. I can do practically anything. It's a miracle cure. It cured my asthma."
— Actress Cloris Leachman

More and more doctors are beginning to recognize the value of fasting to detoxify your physical being. Fasting is God's miracle cleanser.

"Fasting is an effective and safe method of detoxifying the body. Fast regularly and help the body heal itself and stay well."
— *James Balch, M.D.*

"The doctor of the future will give no medicine but will interest his patients in the care of the human frame in diet and in the cause and prevention of disease."
— *Thomas A. Edison*

"To lengthen thy life, lessen thy meals."
— *Benjamin Franklin*

A friend of mine fasts every Wednesday. Many Christians now choose one or two days a week for fasting. People who fast a couple of times a week have healthier, more beautiful complexions. If you're underweight or anemic, fasting can help you put on weight, believe it or not. And if you're overweight, you can be helped as well.

Fasting is not starvation. Fasting is a part of a new way of living. Starvation is the process of dying. You cannot starve your way into good health, but you can fast your way to better health when you fast for the right reasons and for a reasonable period of time.

In reality, fasting itself does not cure anything. It simply gets your body into a position to heal itself by flushing out the causes of your miseries. Your body's responses are merely indicators that the fast is doing its job of cleansing. The elimination of body toxins releases your mind and spirit from physical bondage.

Fasting does not change God; it changes *us* and prepares us for spiritual revelation. It brings us into a spiritual position that amplifies and concentrates the power of God working in us.

CHAPTER 8

YOUR REWARDS FOR FASTING

So far, we've talked about what fasting is, the different types of fasting, the purpose of fasting, and the proper attitudes of fasting. We learned that fasting is abstaining from food or from certain kinds of food, such as your favorite foods. We learned that fasting is a Christian discipline; a practice that a Christian is expected to do. Remember, Jesus said, "*When* you fast," not, "*If* you fast." We also talked about Jesus teaching us to expect a reward from fasting.

This chapter is designed as an exercise for you. When you expect a reward from your fasting, God will get you into a position to receive that reward. I want you to take some time right now to write down the rewards that you are expecting; whatever it is that you want to receive from God for your time of fasting. Be sure to pray first, and ask God for guidance.

1. _____

2. _____

3. _____

4. _____

5. _____

6. _____

7. _____

8. _____

9. _____

10. _____

"And he said unto them, This kind can come forth by nothing, but by prayer and fasting."

— Mark 9:29

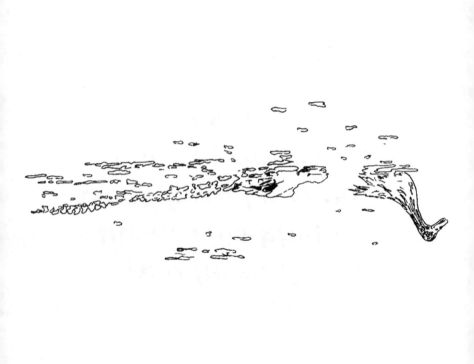

CHAPTER 9

DEFEATING LEVIATHAN

Some years ago I stood in our church narthex talking with a Church of God minister who had been involved with some of the major ministries in this country. He told me about a demonic being that is sometimes loosed against the children of God and the ministries of God. The Bible calls him Leviathan.

Now, I had read about Leviathan in the Bible, but I never knew what it was. I thought it was merely a serpent of some kind — like a sea serpent. As we spoke, this minister told me about a pastor in a major city who had gone through a horrible time of turmoil in his ministry. He said it felt as if he were in the jaws of a monster. That monster would flip him one way, and before he could get out of its grip, the monster would flip him another way. Back and forth he was flung until he was worn out and ready to give up. He wanted to quit and say, "It's all I can take. I can't take any more. It's just too much for me to handle."

That is exactly what Leviathan wants to happen. He wants people of God to give up, to throw in the towel, and say, "That's it."

Let's look at Psalm 74 to learn about this creature, Leviathan, and what it has to do with your time of fasting. I've noticed that Leviathan seems to secretly creep in when a couple of things are happening. First, when there are a lot of people finding salvation, and second, when a church is facing a decision and seeking guidance from God for the proper direction, Leviathan will be lurking to cause problems.

It says in Psalm 74:12-13:

> *"For God is my King of old, working salvation in the midst of the earth. Thou didst divide the sea by thy strength: thou brakest the heads of the dragons in the waters."*

Now notice verse 14:

> *"Thou brakest the heads* (plural) *of the leviathan* (singular) *in pieces, and gavest him*

> *to be meat to the people inhabiting the*
> *wilderness."*

The word "wilderness" represents a time of confusion, of not knowing which way to turn, or where to go. Whenever a child of God or a minister of God or a church that is winning souls faces a wilderness time, you can be sure that Leviathan is nearby ready to strike.

Now read Isaiah 27, because this gives us a little more light on who Leviathan is. We read in verse one:

> *"In that day the Lord with his sore and*
> *great and strong sword shall punish leviathan*
> *the piercing serpent, even leviathan that*
> *crooked serpent: and he shall slay the dragon*
> *that is in the sea."*

Apparently, Leviathan is a powerful demonic spirit under the direct leadership of Satan himself. He is a special creature released against men of God and works of God. He is called a serpent — a crooked serpent. We know as we study the first book of the Bible, Genesis, and the last book of the Bible, Revelation, that Satan himself is called the serpent. He is called the dragon. Here, we find Leviathan called both of those things. In the Hebrew language, the closest word we can find for Leviathan is actually "crocodile."

Now, when my friend from the Church of God was telling me about Leviathan striking major ministries and trying to ruin various works of God around the country, I didn't completely understand it, but it was only to be a year and a half later that Leviathan would strike me and our ministry. I felt like I was a ping-pong ball being battered one way, then the other way. There was so much confusion; I didn't understand what was happening.

Leviathan had come into the church I pastored. I felt like I was in the jaws of a dragon. He threw me one way and then another, thrashing me back and forth. Notice also in Psalm 74, verse 14 it says, "heads," plural. Leviathan seems to have a multitude of heads, and that is why there is so much confusion when Leviathan strikes. He has got one head saying one thing and another head saying another thing and another head saying something else.

I heard so many ridiculous things around our church, but I couldn't pinpoint where they were coming from. I heard rumors about me and about my staff. I heard rumors that we were committing every sin that I ever preached against.

Leviathan had been loosed against us.

At last, I understood firsthand what my friend was talking about when he told me about that particular ministry that had been struck by Leviathan. I finally found out what it was like to be tossed this way, then tossed that way, and then tossed back. I heard terrible lies about myself, and I heard unfounded rumors about my ministry. Suddenly, it seemed like everybody in the world knew more about me than I knew. It was the most awful thing that I have ever experienced in my life.

I began to study crocodiles because I wanted to see if I could find out more about the nature of this hideous, satanic spirit called Leviathan. As I studied, I discovered that people have reported crocodiles up to 30 feet long. However, the average crocodile is really only 12 to 15 feet long, and the largest authentically recorded one was only 23 feet long. This revealed to me that when Leviathan strikes, he always seems bigger than he actually is. Remember, Leviathan has many heads, so when he strikes, there is always confusion.

Another fact about crocodiles is they have a strong, powerful tail. This tail guides them through the water. Crocodiles are found around water and rivers — that is where they like to be. Wherever there is the water of the Holy Spirit, wherever there is a river of life flowing, you will find Leviathan lurking and looking to ruin it somehow. Remember, I said Leviathan strikes where souls are being won.

A crocodile will be very still in the water until a little duck or some other small animal or maybe even a human being comes to the water to get a drink. The crocodile lies motionless in the water, and when he sees his prey, he will slowly, without rippling the water at all, sink down with only his eyes and snout above the water. With his tail moving slowly back and forth propelling him forward, he will silently sneak up on his prey. His prey won't even know what is coming; he is so very quiet. When his victim bows its head to get a drink of water, the crocodile makes a leap, snatching the unwary victim in his mouth. Then he begins to shake his head violently.

You see, there is enough force in a crocodile's jaw to totally crush the animal. But he enjoys torturing that animal by beating it back and forth in the water until the animal gives up fighting and drowns. Then the crocodile eats it. They have been known to eat large animals, such as deer, by just wearing them out.

While I was praying during that terrible time of trial in my ministry, I kept having a picture of a white crocodile-like creature. I would pray and ask,

"God, what is going on?" And I kept getting this vision of a huge, white, crocodile creature.

I asked, "God, what is it?" The word came to me; "Leviathan has been loosed against you." Then I asked, "Well, why is it white?" The Lord responded by saying, "In My Word, you read in the book of Isaiah where it says when I cleanse you from sin, I make your sins as white as snow. In the book of Revelation, when the righteous are standing before the throne, they are clothed in robes of white, which is symbolic of righteousness. Leviathan has come at you in the form of right-ness or righteousness. He is declaring to be right, claiming to be righteous, asserting to stand up for what's right, not caring who he puts in his jaws to ruin."

In my vision, I saw this creature had thick skin. So I asked the Lord, "Why is this white skin on Leviathan so thick?" He said to me, "That's because you can punch him, you can throw rocks at him, you can club him, and it isn't going to bother him one bit. He is not going to go by clubbing. He is not going to go by punching. He is not going to go by speaking to him or commanding him to go. He has thick skin and doesn't care what anybody thinks."

"Howbeit this kind goeth not out but by prayer and fasting."
— *Matthew 17:21*

When we realized what we were up against, we did some fasting in conjunction with much prayer. In a short time, God turned the tables. Leviathan left. As we entered the new year, we found it to be absolutely the greatest year in the history of the church. Everything skyrocketed. Attendance went up over 62 percent. The income went up. Everything in the church grew abundantly. It was almost like there was a release in the church. There were hardly any people hospitalized for any reason. It was the best year that I can ever remember. In fact, I didn't have one nasty "sniper" letter the whole year. Unity, harmony, peace, and success had returned like a dove. The spirit of Leviathan had been broken . . . but only through fasting and prayer.

"And I set my face unto the Lord God, to seek by prayer and supplications, with fasting, and sackcloth, and ashes:"

— Daniel 9:3

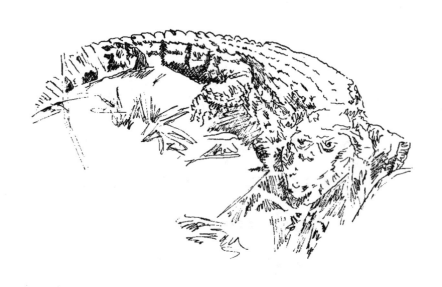

CHAPTER 10

LEVIATHAN'S TAIL

Years ago I met Marlin Lease from Jack Hayford's church, Church on the Way. Jack had told Marlin about the time Leviathan struck his ministry.

I learned more about Leviathan when I attended a national conference for ministers. I heard many renowned men of God share their experiences with Leviathan. They faced exactly the same thing that I faced. As I listened, I thought, "This is the same spirit that came against me." Later I discovered that almost every major ministry in the United States of America has faced Leviathan.

You know, many who have not learned the secret of fasting don't make it out of the jaws of Leviathan. They are defeated and quit.

But Jack Hayford said that when you get out of the jaws of Leviathan, things are going to be good for awhile because Leviathan is moving away. He can't get you in his mouth when he is walking away from you, so things are going to seem pretty good. "But then," Jack continued, "there's something you have to watch out for as Leviathan moves away — his tail. Because as Leviathan, in defeat, walks away from you, he's going to try to get one final blow in with his powerful tail." I believe Jack's word was a word from the Lord, a word of warning not a word of threat. God does not threaten like Satan; God warns. There is a big difference.

You may recall in the book of Revelation how the tail of the dragon knocked the stars out of heaven. He dragged down a third of them with his tail. "If I can't get them with my mouth, I'll get them with my tail," Leviathan says.

I believe that through fasting and prayer you can avoid the swishing tail of Leviathan. You may feel a little draft go over your head, but that is as close as he is going to get; because when you fast, you are entering into dynamic spiritual warfare. In fasting and prayer, you will gain a concentrated, intensified power from God and protection all around you.

FASTING IS THE SECRET WEAPON OF SPIRITUAL WARFARE

Whenever our church sends out a young minister to plant a new church in another community, we ask that his first action be to fast for at least ten days. Fasting will help fine tune his spiritual senses, making it easy for him to identify any of Satan's strongholds in that city, including Leviathan. Fasting seems to sensitize his discernment, helping him to understand the evil principalities and territorial spirits in the area.

> *"For we wrestle not against flesh and blood, but against principalities, against powers, against the rulers of the darkness of this world, against spiritual wickedness in high places."*
>
> — *Ephesians 6:12*

Once recognized, these usurping, evil beings can be dealt with powerfully. You can't deal with an enemy you don't recognize. Satan's work is undercover work; it is secretive, deceptive, and hidden. That is why fasting is critical to beginning a new work in a city or community. We have learned that ministers who have fasted first become successful and fruitful quickly. Those who bypass this step seem to struggle with the same problems year after year.

Fasting is the secret weapon in our arsenal of spiritual artillery.

We are going to see hundreds of thousands of people coming to Christ in the days ahead. We are going to see marvelous, spectacular growth, not only in our church, but also in our personal lives. We need to launch out into the deep and extend our vision. God has big plans for you and me.

This revival is going to ripple around the world. Leviathan can't stop it. There are too many Christians learning that fasting is the secret weapon.

CHAPTER 11

PROMISED BENEFITS FROM ISAIAH 58

Now let's look again at Isaiah 58 to find the promises to the person who makes regular fasting a way of life.

In verse 6 it says, "*Is not this the fast that I have chosen? to loose the bands of wickedness . . .*". We are going to see bands of wickedness loosed, torn off, undone. The word "bands" actually means fetters; things that hold people back.

THINGS THAT HOLD YOU BACK

Have you ever felt held back for some reason? Has something held you back from advancing and moving ahead? I promise you, on the basis of Isaiah 58, that if you get involved in fasting, those bands of wickedness, those fetters, whatever it is that has been holding you back, are going to be loosed, and your life will advance.

HEAVY BURDENS VANISH

Also look at verse 6 where it says, *"and undo the heavy burdens . . ."*. Heavy burdens are going to be lifted. Do you know what "undo" means in the Hebrew? It means to violently shake off. Many people are carrying burdens that God never intended for them to carry. They are going to be undone — shaken off — as a result of fasting.

ARE YOU "CRACKING UP?"

In verse 6, it also says, *"and to let the oppressed go free . . ."*. The word "oppressed" in the original language means discouraged, bruised, crushed, hurt. It actually has a literal meaning which, in a picture, is a vase cracked in pieces. The word means "cracking up." The promise is that those who are "cracking up" are going to go free.

Have you ever felt like you were cracking up?

Do you know there are people around you who really hurt? They are bruised. They are wounded. They are what we call the "walking wounded."

They are going to be set free because of your fasting for them!

The Bible says God anointed Jesus of Nazareth who went about doing good and healing all that were "cracking up," oppressed by the devil. The devil can oppress people to where they think they are cracking up. But, through your fasting, they are going to be set free! We need to humble ourselves and put ourselves into a position where God can use us to heal the oppressed and bind up the broken hearted.

HABITS WILL BE BROKEN

Again, refer to Isaiah 58, verse 6: *"ye break every yoke..."*. A yoke is a habit, a thing that you just cannot seem to break.

I have known people who have had the nicotine habit, but after three days of fasting, it was gone. Somebody said to me after a service, "I want you to pray that I'll quit smoking." I said, "You fast for three days. Just drink water and you're not going to want a cigarette. You won't want one. You're going to be delivered. That yoke is going to be broken. I guarantee it." Breaking habits is part of the Christian discipline called fasting.

I read about a man who was not Spirit-filled, and he did not believe in speaking in tongues. Then he read about fasting. He was a born-again Christian, but he had a problem with cigarettes. He fasted for a few days; then all of a sudden, he did not want cigarettes anymore. While he was praying, something bubbly began to rise up in his belly. Out of his mouth came words he had never learned with his intellect, and suddenly, he was speaking in tongues. He was delivered from tobacco and received the baptism of the Holy Spirit at the same time as a result of fasting.

Your yokes will be broken by fasting.

YOU CAN GIVE TO THE POOR

Verse 7 says, *"Is it not to deal thy bread to the hungry, and that thou bring the poor that are cast out into thy house? when thou seest the naked, that thou cover him . . .".* You are going to save a little money by fasting. When you are not buying food, what do you think you are supposed to do with that money? "Oh boy, I have more money to play pinball machines," you say. That is not what the money is for. It is so you can feed the hungry. Have you ever watched those poor, little kids on television and said, "Oh, I just wish I had $15 to send to them!" Here is your opportunity. Fast a few meals. That will save you $15. You can send it in to the poor. This is the fast God has chosen. All these wonderful benefits are going to take place when you do it God's way.

REVELATION KNOWLEDGE

Verse 8 says, *"Then shall thy light break forth as the morning . . .".* What does this mean? Well, what do you call morning light? Dawn. Have you ever said, "Oh, it just dawned on me"?

Have you ever been reading the Bible and suddenly something dawns on you? We call that revelation. You are going to receive revelation from God during your time of fasting. Daniel was fasting and received revelation from God. You will enjoy more frequent and more intense revelation from God as a result of fasting.

Martin Luther, the man who translated the Bible from Hebrew and Greek into the German language, fasted and prayed. He probably prayed, "God, help me. I don't know how to do this. I need your help in translating this Bible." He was fasting during every word he translated. To this very day, Luther's translation is still the most accurate, the most excellent, and the highest quality translation there is in the German language. It is still used by the German people today because of its accuracy.

Revelation comes during times of fasting. It is amazing how ordinary people can receive heaven-sent ideas that can catapult them ahead in businesses and ministries.

I read about a pastor that could never understand the book of Revelation. It really frustrated him because he wanted to teach his people about Bible prophecy, but he could not even understand it himself. You cannot teach something you do not understand yourself. So he began to fast. All of a sudden, God unlocked his understanding to the book of Revelation. He was able to teach it to his people, and they were all excited and happy about the second coming of Jesus. He has been able to understand Bible prophecy ever since. Revelation will come to you.

HEALTH RETURNS QUICKLY

Verse 8 also says, *"and thine health shall spring forth speedily."* "Well," someone says, "it might be God's will for me to mend slowly." No, that is not what the Bible says. It says, through fasting, your health will spring forth speedily.

How may teenagers have complexion problems? It has been discovered that if teenagers fast a couple of days a week, their complexion problem will take care of itself. They will not have to rub that gooey stuff on every night.

I told my daughter when she was four years old, "Honey, you've got to quit eating so much chocolate because it'll give you pimples." She would take a little drink of chocolate milk and then run to look in the mirror to see if any pimples came. When they didn't, she would take another little drink of chocolate milk, run and look, then feel her face. "Are they there yet?" she asked. She planned to drink chocolate milk just until the sign of a pimple arrived, and then she was going to quit.

Many doctors are now encouraging their patients to fast once a week because they see the speedy physical results of fasting. Fasting will benefit you spiritually, mentally, and physically. Your health will spring forth speedily. Fasting will benefit you in every way.

I read about a sickly man who was underweight. He began to fast and lost 16 pounds. He kept fasting. Soon he began to put on weight until he gained 29 pounds. He went right up to the weight that was desirable for his body size and then quit fasting. His anemic condition left, and he was completely healed and at the ideal weight. Most of us do not have that problem. Most of us have that other problem (I think in the Greek language, it's called being *fat*. Or is that the Hebrew?). Fasting will help you either way.

DIVINE PROTECTION

Still from Isaiah 58, verse 8 says, *"thy righteousness shall go before thee . . . ".* In other words, you are going to have a shield in front of you. Then it says, *"the glory of the Lord shall be thy rereward,"* or rear guard. The glory of the Lord is going to guard you. There will be no sneak attacks because the glory of the Lord is going to be following you around everywhere you go. *"Then shalt thou call, and the Lord shall answer; thou shalt cry, and He shall say, Here I am."* I like the Living Bible paraphrase. It says, "Your prayers have been answered speedily." Do you think God answers prayer quickly now? Wait until you practice fasting. Watch how quickly those prayers are answered!

SUCCESS IS YOURS

Verse 10 says, *"And if thou draw out thy soul to the hungry, and satisfy the afflicted soul; then shall thy light rise in obscurity, and thy darkness be as the noonday . . . ".* Do you know what that means? It means you are going to become very successful. You will simply rise out of obscurity and become a real somebody.

Jerry Prevell went to professional counselors to be tested to find out what he would be good at. The counselors examined his skills and said, "Well, you'd be good at engineering." He said, "I kind of thought that God called me to the ministry." The job counselors said, "Forget it. You don't have what it takes to be a minister. Go into engineering. Do yourself a favor."

So he started into engineering college. He was in college for about three years, but the call of God would not leave him. He left college, went into the ministry, and fasted because he didn't know what to do. Out of obscurity, Jerry Prevell, from being an unknown, rose to become a very successful pastor of the largest church in Anchorage, Alaska. The professional people said, "No way. You're not cut out for it." Yet through fasting and prayer, God took Jerry and lifted him from obscurity to success.

DIVINE GUIDANCE

Verse 11 says, *"And the Lord shall guide thee continually . . .".* You will not have to get on the phone and call your friend and say, "I just don't know what to do." Instead, God will be guiding you continually.

You are going to receive some guidance during your time of fasting, or shortly thereafter. You are going to receive direction for your life. You will not have to say, "I don't know what I'm going to do. What should I do?" God will be right there telling you what to do! He promised to guide us, not just some of the time, but continually, over and over again. The steps of a good person are ordered by the Lord. Step by step, He will show you what to do.

SUPERNATURAL SUPPLY

Verse 11 also says, *"and satisfy thy soul in drought, and make fat thy bones: and thou shalt be like a watered garden, and like a spring of water, whose waters fail not."* In other words, it does not matter what the economic conditions of the world are; you are going to have all you need. Your needs are going to be supplied no matter what the situation is.

Dan Rather, or some other newscaster, can tell you that a depression is coming, the stock market is expected to drop, banks are closing (and it's probably your bank), and the S&L's are going out of business. They will say people are in lines three miles long waiting to get their money out. Don't worry — the Bible says *your* needs are going to be met. God is going to provide for *you*.

FROM DESOLATION TO GLORY

Finally, in verse 12, it says, *"And they that shall be of thee shall build the old waste places: thou shalt raise up the foundations of many generations; and thou shalt be called, The repairer of the breach, The restorer of paths to dwell in."* As a result of fasting, wastelands will turn into fruitful orchards.

As a church, we took 43 acres of desolate land on Creyts Road, in Lansing, Michigan, and devised a master plan for that site. We took a desolate piece of land and turned it into an orchard where spiritual fruit is growing; an international outreach center, printing headquarters, a television production center, a youth action center, and more.

I know of a man that took a bar and nightclub and turned it into a church. I would say that a bar is a pretty desolate wasteland, wouldn't you? Yes, he caught lots of criticism at first because six nights a week it was still a bar and nightclub. He was only renting it as a church on Sundays.

That church grew. The income went up, and they were able to buy the nightclub and turn it into a church seven days a week. Praise God!

This verse means you will be able to take desolate land and turn it into fruitful orchards. I believe it is talking about soulwinning; taking desolate, barren lives destroyed by drugs, alcohol, illicit sex, and the other problems that are permeating our society today and turning them into fruitful orchards for God. Fasting can take people whose lives are ruined by problems and bring them into victory. Their lives will reflect His glory.

Let's review the promises found in Isaiah 58 for the Christian who practices fasting:

1. You'll be released from what's holding you back.
2. Heavy burdens will be broken.
3. You will have freedom from discouragement and wounds.
4. Bad habits will be broken.
5. The hungry will be fed.
6. Divine revelation will come to you.
7. Your health will spring forth speedily.
8. God's glory will guard your life.
9. Prayers will be answered speedily.
10. You will rise out of obscurity to prominence.
11. The Lord Himself will guide you continually.
12. Your needs will all be met regardless of economic conditions.
13. Desolation will turn into high production.

These are just the promises in Isaiah 58. Throughout the Bible, you'll read of other benefits to fasting. Who wouldn't want to fast for three days, seven days, ten days, or even forty days with these great benefits?

CHAPTER 12

CHOOSE YOUR PLAN, AND TAKE ACTION

After reading this book on fasting, I trust you are ready to spring into a season of fasting yourself. I have done my best to motivate and inspire you to fast without wearing you out with unnecessary verbiage and clutter.

In this chapter, I want to give you some ideas for planning regular times of fasting throughout the year. Remember, if you have some physical condition that you are concerned about, please consult an enlightened health care professional before beginning an extended fast. Some folks who cannot fast for long periods of time can simply abstain from one meal a day, for example, or one meal a day for two or more days.

Prepare for your fast by making a firm commitment to stick to it. Don't listen to your screaming appetite. Appetite is not the same as hunger. True hunger doesn't come until after about 40 days of fasting. You recall, after Jesus fasted 40 days, he was hungry. That was true hunger not simply appetite crying out to be fed. You can be almost sure that after just a few hours, your appetite will be crying and whining, wanting to be fed. That is why you need to make a quality commitment to fast — to bring your body into subjection to your will.

> *"But I keep under my body, and bring it into subjection: lest that by any means, when I have preached to others, I myself should be a castaway."*
> — *I Corinthians 9:27*

THE PREPARATION

First, prepare for your fast. Next, determine your reward. Now don't misunderstand; you are not going to get $6 million from God just because you fasted six days. But, if you need $6 million to advance your gospel ministry, don't be afraid to ask God for it. God is more willing to give good things to His children than His children are willing to believe Him for. Remember, the main goal of fasting is to position yourself to hear from God and draw closer to Him — to experience His presence. That is what we really need.

DETERMINING YOUR REWARD

In determining your reward, remember Jesus said, secret seeking brings open reward. Think of loved ones that need a relationship with God. Name as your reward their salvation. Think of those who are afflicted and sick. Name "deliverance" for them as your reward. How about your neighbors who have no relationship to Christ or to His church. Name "salvation" as their reward. What about your particular needs for guidance? Write them down, and be specific. What are the questions you would like God to answer? What are your personal needs, your desires? Write them all down. Ask God to reward your fasting. You must have specific rewards written out to effectively fast for a desired result. Go back to Chapter 8 of this book to write down your fasting rewards.

PRAYER

Next, it is important to do extra praying during times of fasting. At our church, there are all kinds of opportunities for prayer involvement: daily prayer (early morning, noon, and afternoon), 120 prayer meetings, Fresh Fire prayer meetings, Revival Rally prayer meetings, back room intercessory prayer meetings, home prayer meetings, and others. Some way, somehow, get involved in a weekly prayer meeting during your time of fasting.

Also, you will want to invest the time that you would normally be eating as time in prayer. Instead of eating, you will be praying. Pray for others. Here is a good plan to stretch your vision. Pray for a person or family who lives across the street from you, behind you, and on each side of you. Pray for them daily, mentioning them to God. If you are a student, pray for the classmates who sit in front of you, behind you, and on each side of you. Ask God to move mightily in their lives and give you favor with them. Ask God for revelation on how you might express some encouraging, Holy Spirit-led words to them.

Now, let's select a plan for fasting.

I like to begin the new year with a 40 day concentrated, corporate fast. To be honest, I have never fasted completely for the 40 days. I have done a Daniel fast for over forty days. The longest I have totally abstained from food, to date, was seven days. That is okay. As you study church history, you find that most times of fasting were short. Only under unusual and extraordinary circumstances did people fast for 40 days. Yet, you can fast forty days this way:

☑ PLAN A - Fast completely for three days, drinking only distilled water. After that, drink juices for a few days, then eat only fruits and vegetables for the remaining days. (This is called a "Daniel Fast.")

☑ PLAN B - Fast completely for seven days, drinking only distilled water. After that, drink juices for a few days, then "Daniel Fast" for the remainder of the days.

☑ PLAN C - Fast one designated day per week for a whole year. That's 52 days!

☑ PLAN D - Fast two designated days a week for a whole year. That's 104 days!

☑ PLAN E - Fast three to seven days every three months, plus once a week.

☑ PLAN F - Skip one or two meals on designated days each week.

☑ PLAN G - Do a "Daniel Fast" for as many days as God directs. This means consuming distilled water, juices, vegetables, and fruits only. Perhaps you can designate one day a week as your "meat day" and stay on the "Daniel Fast" for the other days.

DEVELOP YOUR OWN PLAN

You can also develop your own plan for fasting as it fits your schedule and life-style. As I said in an earlier chapter, fasting is not to be a legalistic practice but a body cleansing, spiritually rejuvenating practice. You should expect marvelous rewards.

A FINAL WORD OF ENCOURAGEMENT

I must warn you. As you fast, you will notice impurities and toxins coming out of your body in various ways. This cleansing process sometimes causes physical responses. Do not let them deter you. They will pass if you give it enough time. If you are doing a total fast (distilled water only), after about three days you may notice that you are not hungry at all. You may find yourself with amazing bursts of energy. However, if you eat, even vitamins or juices, your appetite will stay active, and you will experience hunger pains throughout your time of fasting.

Just as the body cleanses itself during personal fasting, a church body cleanses itself during corporate fasting. Attitudes will manifest. Those who are not really "on the team" will reveal themselves. It is painfully amazing, and healthy for a church, so do not worry about it. It is only a God-given sifting, or pruning, which will bring the church to greater productivity and fruitfulness.

And remember, quite often the major benefits of fasting come after the fast is complete. That is why you need to make your commitment and stick to it.

Get ready for a new experience that will lead you to greater revelation and a closer relationship with Jesus than you ever knew you could have. Prepare for miracles! Gear up for the best year of your life as answers to your prayers come speedily and good health springs forth like a fresh river.

Keep your focus on the benefits.

Once again . . . Happy Fasting!

"But as for me, when they were sick, my clothing was sackcloth: I humbled my soul with fasting; and my prayer returned into mine own bosom."

— Psalm 35:13

Now it's up to You

If you have been moved by the Holy Spirit to participate in the spiritual discipline of fasting, please let me know. I want to hear from you. Simply tear out this page (or make a photocopy), and send it to me. I want to pray for you during your time of fasting. Write, or fax me at:

Dave Williams
202 S. Creyts Road
Lansing, MI 48917-8229
Fax: (517) 321-6332

☑ Yes, Pastor Dave. I'll join you in fasting.

I'll fast _____ meal(s) per day for ____ days.
I'll fast _____ days each week for ____ weeks.
I'll fast this way:

_____

_____

Here are the "rewards" I need from God:

_____

_____

_____

Please Pray for:

_____

_____

My Name: _____
My Address: _____
City: _____ State: _____ Zip: _____
Phone: _____ Fax: _____
Email: _____

Published by

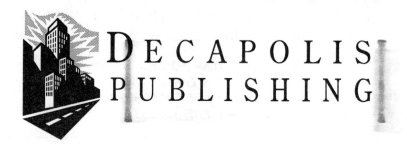

DECAPOLIS
PUBLISHING

202 SOUTH CREYTS ROAD
LANSING, MI 48917-9284

For a catalog of products
write to the above address, or call:

1-800-888-7284

or
1-517-321-2780

For Your Spiritual Growth

We all need help on our spiritual journey. These books will encourage you, and give you guidance as you seek to draw close to Jesus, and learn of Him. Prepare yourself for fantastic growth!

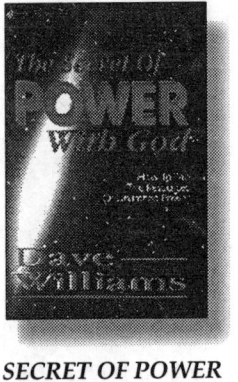

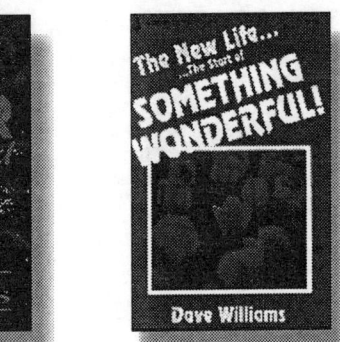

BE A HIGH PER-FORMANCE BELIEVER
Pour in the nine spiritual additives for real power in your Christian life.

SECRET OF POWER WITH GOD
Tap into the real power with God, the power of prayer. It will change your life!

THE NEW LIFE . . .
You can get off to a great start on your exciting life with Jesus! Prepare for something wonderful.

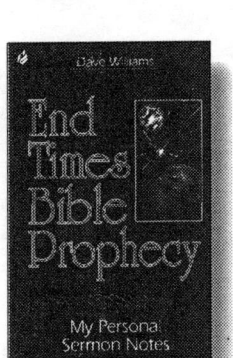

GIFTS OF THE HOLY SPIRIT
Reach beyond this natural world, into the creative supernatural realm of God's gifts and power.

END TIMES BIBLE PROPHECY
Watch as events God spoke about thousands of years ago unfold to show us the time of Christ's return.

THE AIDS PLAGUE
Is there hope? Yes, but only Jesus can bring anyone a total and lasting cure to AIDS. But we must diligently follow His prescription.

These and other books available from Dave Williams and:

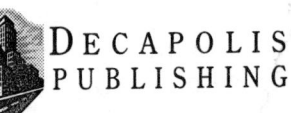

DECAPOLIS PUBLISHING

For Your Successful Life

These video cassettes will give you successful principles to apply to your whole life. Each a different topic, and each a fantastic teaching of how living by God's word can give you total success!

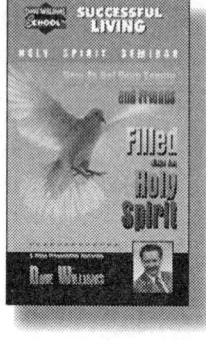

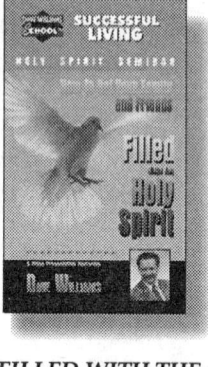

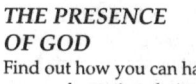

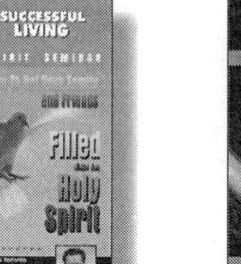

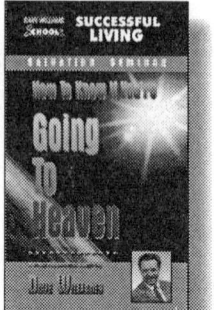

THE PRESENCE OF GOD
Find out how you can have a more dynamic relationship with the Holy Spirit.

FILLED WITH THE HOLY SPIRIT
You can rejoice and share with others in this wonderful experience of God.

HOW TO KNOW IF YOU'RE GOING TO HEAVEN
You can be sure of your eternal destination!

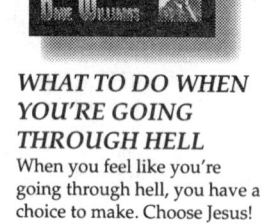

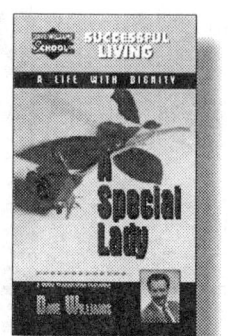

WHAT TO DO WHEN YOU'RE GOING THROUGH HELL
When you feel like you're going through hell, you have a choice to make. Choose Jesus!

SPECIAL LADY
If you feel used and abused, this video will show you how you really are in the eyes of Jesus. You are special!

These and other videos available from Dave Williams and:

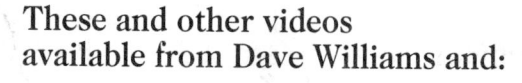

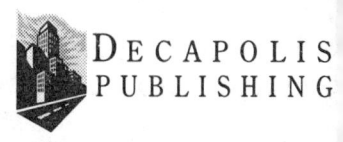

DECAPOLIS
PUBLISHING